Pre-Parental Workbook:

Preparing Yourself, Your Relationship and Your Family for Having a Baby

By Chandra Heath,
Licensed Marriage and Family Therapist

Dedication

To my husband for being so supportive and such a wonderful father.

ISBN-13: 978-1466264168

ISBN-10: 1466264160

Edited by Susan E. Lindsey, Savvy Communication LLC, Louisville, KY

Photography by Melissa Mann Bean, Mann Photography, melissamannphotography.com

Photograph page 8 - digital skillet (istockphoto.com)

Photograph page 14 - Felix Mizioznikov (istockphoto.com)

Photograph page 24 - Juan Monino (istockphoto.com)

Photograph page 26 - Daniel Laflor (istockphoto.com)

Creative Services by bluegrasscreative.com

Introduction

Research has suggested that of all the couples who marry, about 50 percent will divorce. Many of these couples will do so within the first five to seven years of marriage. According to family studies, after the couple begins their family, marital satisfaction begins to decrease. Adding to the stress of a new baby, are changes in family dynamics, and responsibilities and priorities. Preparing for these changes, honest communication, and realistic expectations may decrease the divorce rate, and infant abuse, and increase marital or relational satisfaction.

When a relationship begins to experience stress, the stress is carried over into other areas of life: work, family, friends, and so on. Soon, stress begins to encompass most of the areas of life, including one's thought processes. Often this level of stress can be prevented if we are willing to work through our emotions and seek help from others.

Sadly, sometimes the stress level can turn violent (intentionally or unintentionally) and is typically focused on the ones we love. When we react based on our emotions, we put ourselves and others in danger. Though I would like to think that no one would intentionally hurt a baby, the truth is, many times, the baby in the family tends to be the focus of aggression that results in major injuries.

Taking preventive measures is the key to preserving relationships, and keeping you and your family safe. This workbook is designed to be a tool to help you achieve these goals.

What is a Partner?

A partner is anyone helping you with your baby on a consistent basis. This could be, but is not limited to: spouse, family member, friend, roommate or significant other.

Before You Start

During your discussion times with your partner, you may experience some undesirable emotions. I encourage you to be open and honest with each other. Sometimes, outside help is needed to work through struggles from the past or present. This help may be in the form of a mentor couple, support group, or a professional counselor. Do not hesitate to seek outside help should you feel you or your family need it.

Chapter 1: Communication and Honesty

Sometimes it is difficult to be honest about how you are truly feeling. However, when we suppress how we feel about something, we begin to experience undesirable emotions. If these emotions persist, often they resurface with more intensity than when we first experienced them. These emotions are then typically expressed verbally and/or physically. To keep ourselves and others safe, it is vital that we learn to communicate effectively, and be honest with ourselves about how we truly feel.

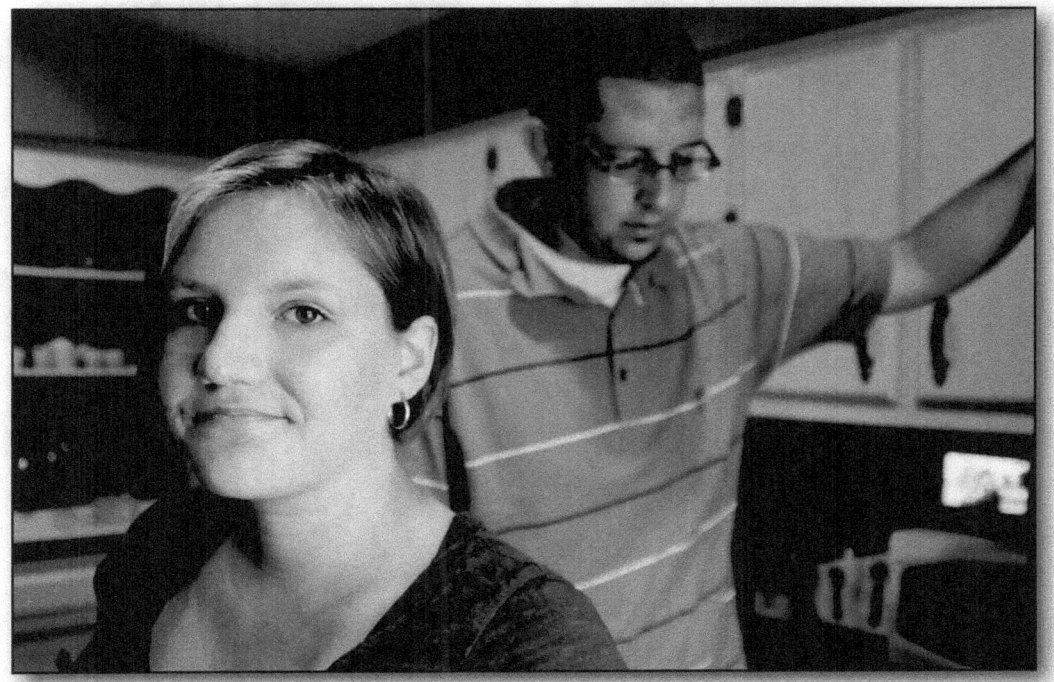

1. What are some barriers from the past and present that prevent you from being open about your feelings?

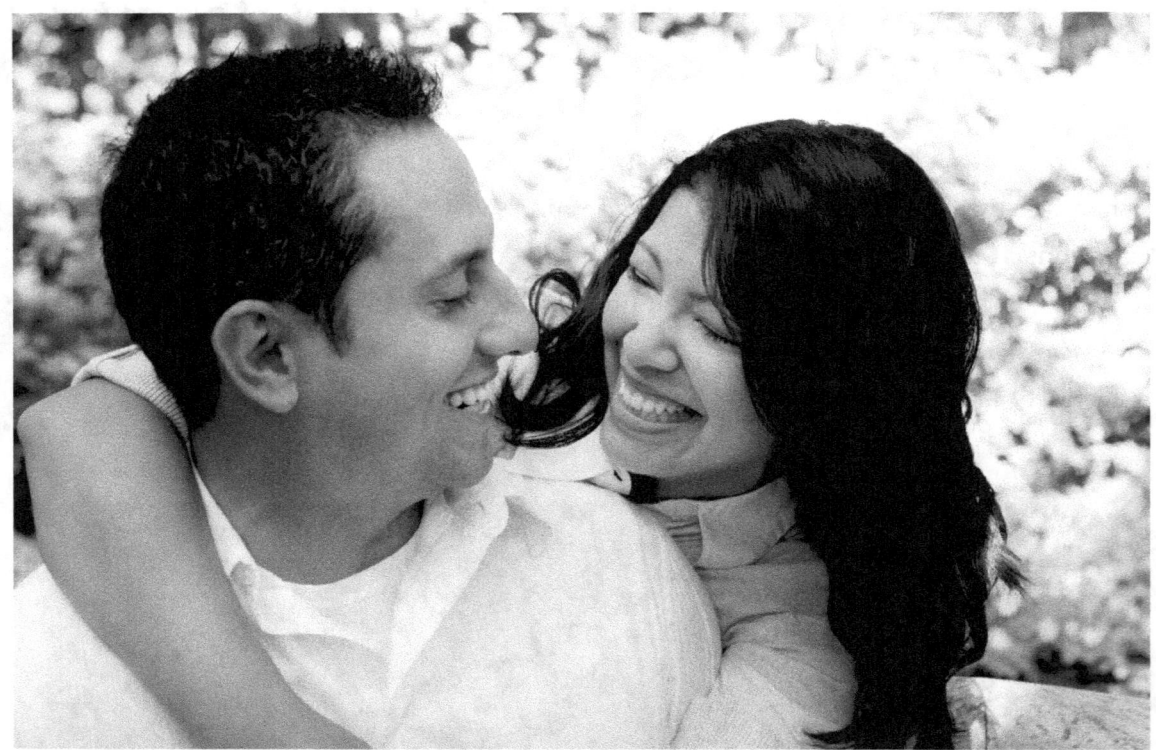

2. Do you suppress your feelings? If so, what do you feel causes you to suppress your feelings?

3. Do you struggle with expressing your negative feelings in a non-hurtful way (emotionally, physically or verbally)?

4. What fears do you have about expressing your feelings to your partner?

5. How can your partner help you to effectively communicate (be open minded, refrain from judgment, give you their sole attention, etc.)?

6. Is there any anger, fear, or hurt that you need to discuss with your partner so you can resolve it, and release undesirable emotions?

Chapter 2: Pregnancy and Finances

Many factors need to be considered when deciding to have a child. Being open and honest when talking about these factors is key to starting this new life together.

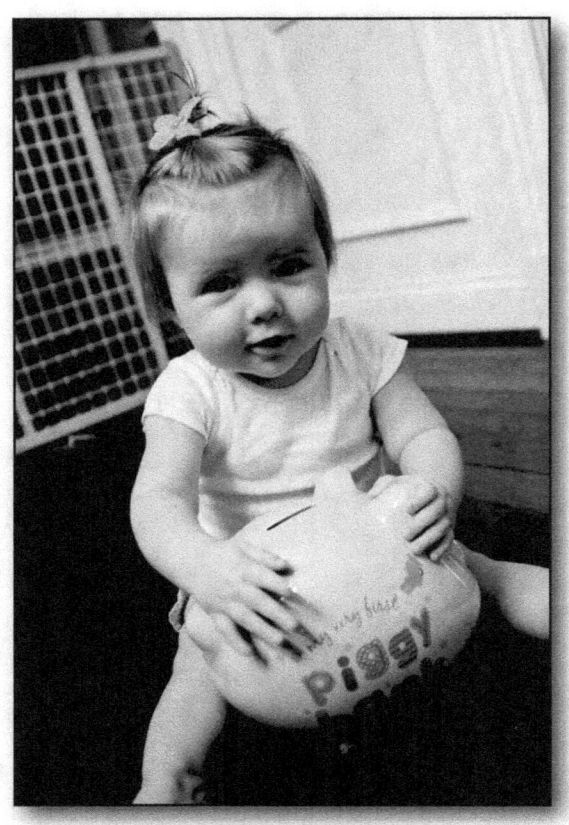

The following questions deal with topics that you might want to discuss before you try to get pregnant.

1. How do you feel about bringing a baby into your relationship or family? Do you feel ready? What concerns do you have?

2. How will your work schedules fit with having a baby? Are there expectations for yourself or your partner to change work schedules or stay at home with the baby?

I know that the next few questions may seem to focus on money, but money is one of the main causes of relationships ending. Please take some time to discuss the following questions, and if needed, take time to do some research and examine your finances.

3. Do you feel that you can meet the financial needs of your family if there is a new baby? You may want to consider taking a trip to the grocery store to inquire about the prices of items such as formula, diapers, and other baby essentials.

4. How much will it cost to add a dependent to your health insurance plan?

5. What is the average cost of child care in your area? You may want to call daycare centers, talk to private childcare providers, or talk with friends who use baby sitters or daycare centers.

Sometimes pregnancies are not planned. Discussing the relevant topics above can still be helpful to be prepared. If you do not feel you are ready to have a baby, please discuss the following. Remember to be open and honest.

6. What are the community resources available for me/us to help as I/we go through pregnancy (support, finances, insurance, etc.)?

7. What steps do I need to take to obtain support from community or government agencies?

8. Should I/we consider putting the baby up for adoption?

Chapter 3: When to Tell

Finding out you are going to have a baby can be very exciting. Sometimes, when people find out they are having a baby, they want to tell everyone immediately. Other people want to keep it a secret until they are months into the pregnancy.

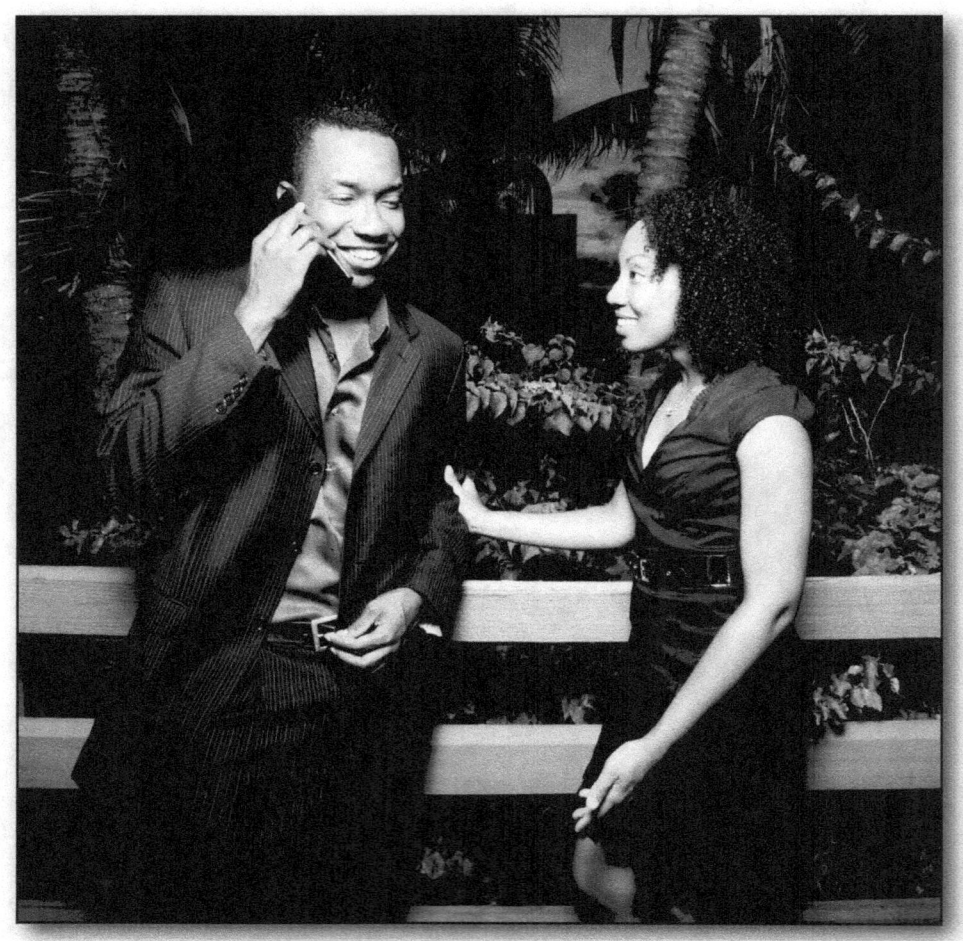

1. How long do you want to wait to tell others about your pregnancy?

2. Are there certain people who you want to tell(so they can provide support) before your news becomes public?

3. If you decide to tell a few people your "secret," are you concerned any of them cannot keep the news to themselves?

4. You may want to compose a list of people you would like to tell and discuss your list with your partner.

Chapter 4: Miscarriages

One reason people refrain from telling others about a pregnancy is the risk of having a miscarriage. This is not a topic that many people trying to have a baby like to discuss, but it's better to be prepared in case something like that does happen.

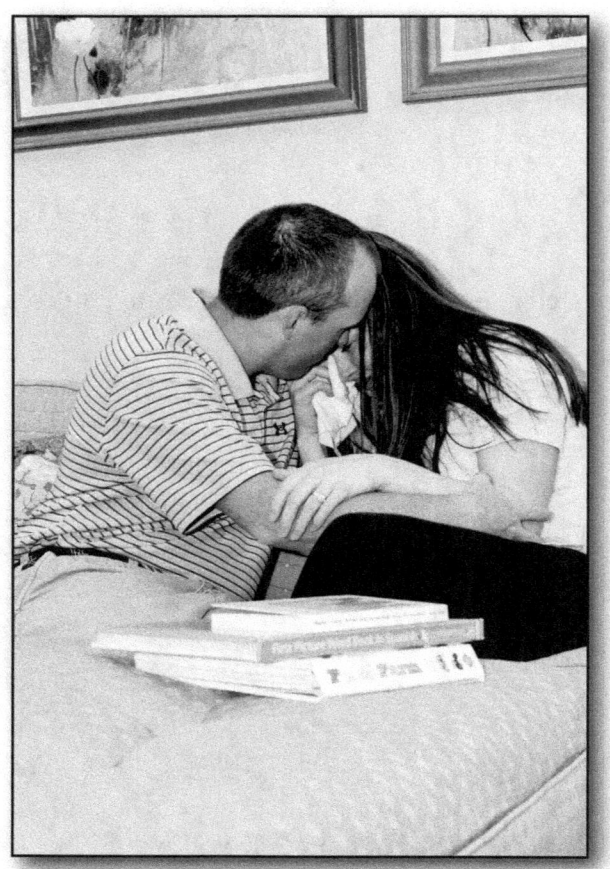

This section can also be helpful if you have experienced a miscarriage in the past.

1. Do either of you have fears of having a miscarriage?

2. If you have had a miscarriage, are you experiencing negative feelings about the miscarriage (guilt, anger, etc.), how are you reacting to your emotions? How do you plan on managing your negative emotions?

3. Are you and your partner experiencing different feelings about the miscarriage or even the topic of miscarriage? Take some time to talk about how you experienced the miscarriage, how you both emotionally reacted to it, or the different feelings you have about the topic of miscarriages. Do not be surprised if you have different perspectives. Be open to what each other has to say.

4. Are you open to talking with family or friends if you should experience a miscarriage or if you have experienced one in the past? Do you feel you have a good support system? If you do not, how could you develop a support system (community resources, church, friends, family, etc.)?

Chapter 5: Mood Swings

As a woman moves further along in pregnancy, emotions can run high and feelings on both sides can become hurt. Changes in moods are pretty much a given, but learning how to deal with these changes can help prevent hurt.

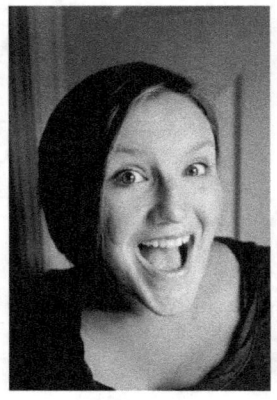 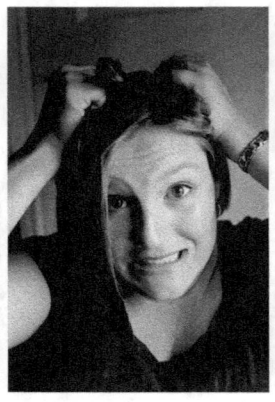 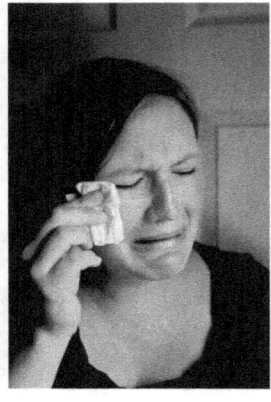 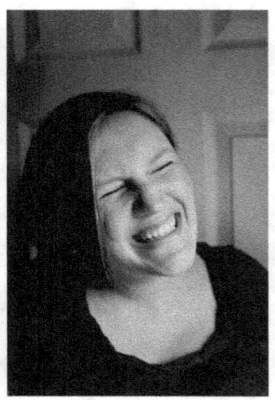

1. How have or how do you plan to deal with changes in mood?

2. What are some cues you can give to each other to signal that the mood changes are becoming hurtful?

3. Discuss if/how your relationship has changed due to changes in moods.

4. Discuss what you need from your partner to get through this difficult time of negative emotions (i.e. alone time, sensitivity, comfort, etc.).

Chapter 6: The Baby's Gender

Deciding to find out if you are having a boy or a girl can be very exciting. It can also be very exciting to find out on the day of delivery.

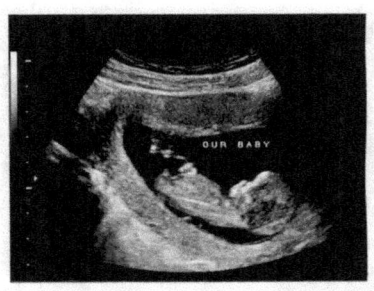

1.Do you want to find out the gender of your baby by ultrasound or by delivery?

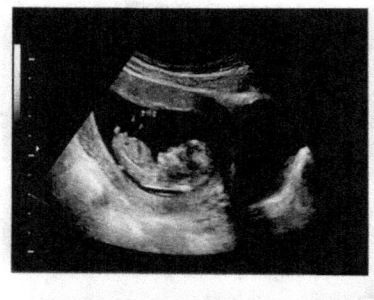

2.If you find out the gender of your baby, do you want to tell others or keep it a secret?

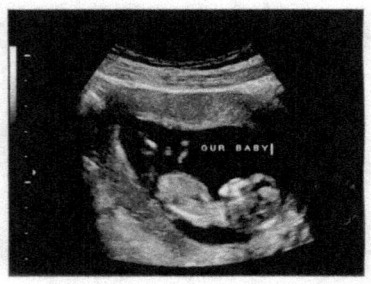

Many times, people ask expectant parents, "Do you want a girl or a boy?" The typical response is something like this: "I don't care about the gender, just as long as the baby is healthy." I am sure that for some people, that is true, but for another group, it is not. Sometimes, deep down, there may be a very strong desire for a baby of a specific gender. If this desire is not discussed, the moment you find out the gender can be a very disappointing time, and it can even ruin the news for your partner.

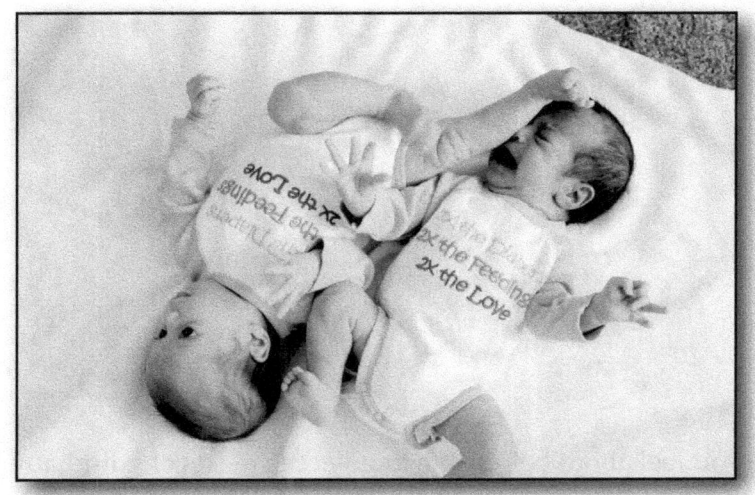

3. Take some time to talk honestly about your desire for your baby to be a specific gender.

4. Discuss how you would initially feel if you do not get the gender you hope for.

5. Do you have negative feelings about your partner's reaction?

6. How do you feel about being able to meet the needs of your baby based on either gender?

Chapter 7: Illnesses Detected in the Womb

At some point in your pregnancy, you will be given the option to take tests to determine the health of your baby. These tests detect serious illnesses and birth defects.

1. Do you want to know if your baby has a serious illness or birth defect?

2. Do you and your partner agree on taking the test or not taking the test?

3. If your baby were to have a serious illness or birth defect, does that change your desire to have a baby? If it does, do you plan on keeping the baby?

If your baby should have a serious illness or birth defect, it may be helpful to do some research about the illness or defect. You might also want to seek out parent support groups or counseling.

Chapter 8: Names

Deciding on a name can be a very fun time for a couple, but it can also be a very stressful time.

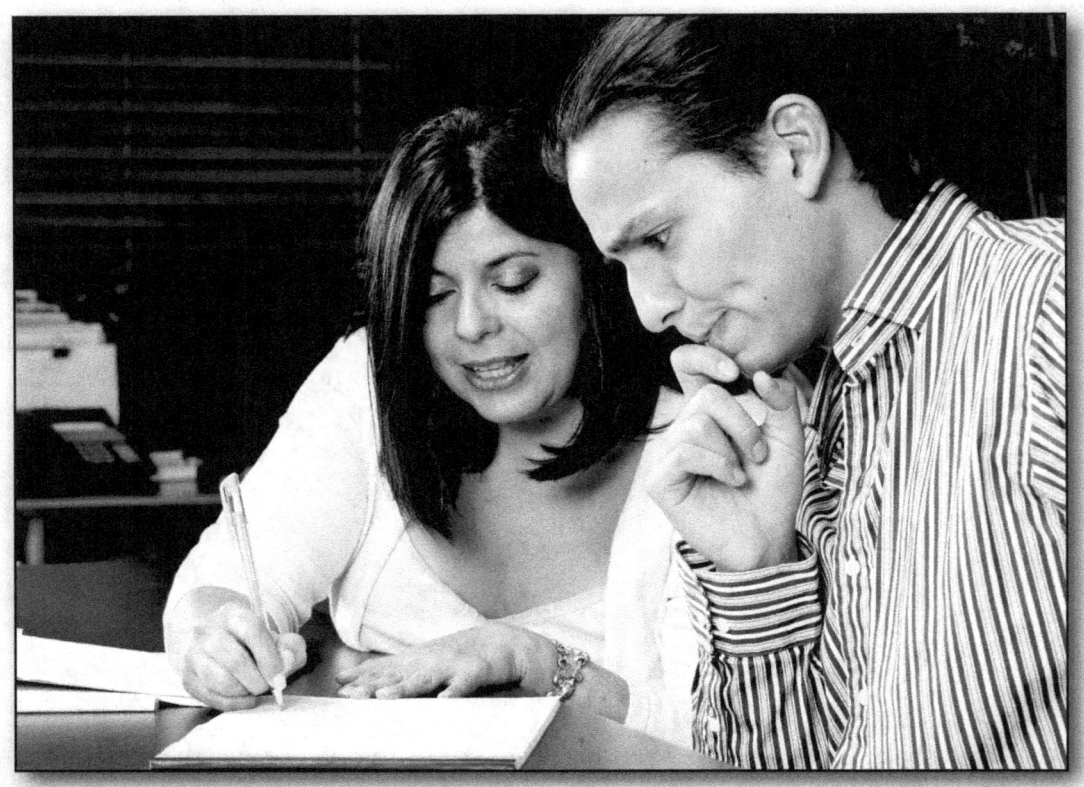

1. What names do each of you like for your baby?

2. How will you compromise on a name?

3. Is there pressure from outsiders causing stress over naming the baby?

4. Do we tell others the baby's name in advance of the birth?

5. How will we respond if others are negative about our baby's name?

Chapter 9: Baby Items

Some couples feel that they need all new items for their child, while some couples are more comfortable borrowing or using secondhand items. Regardless, there are some essentials that the baby will need.

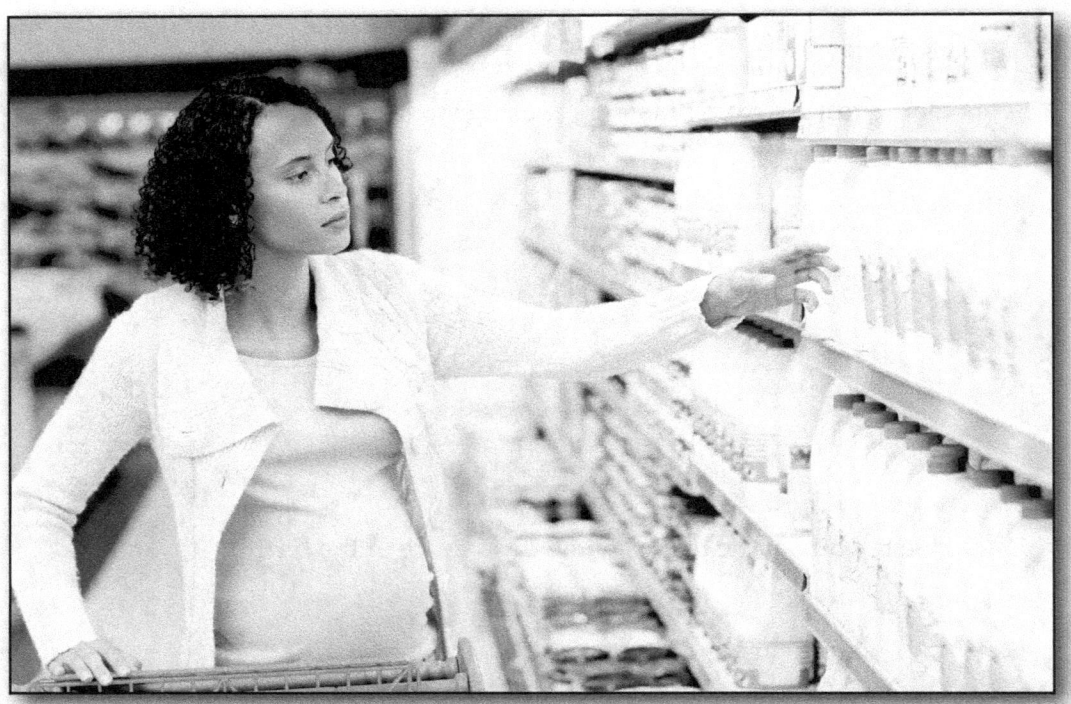

1.   Do we use new, borrowed or used items (or a combination)?

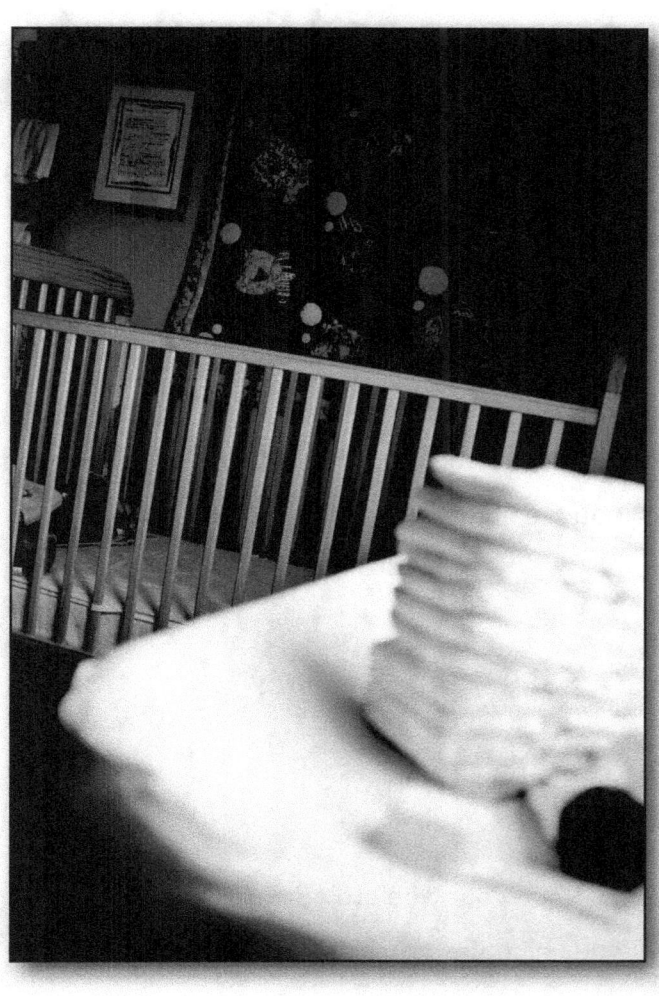

2. Do we want to talk to our friends or family members who have had children to find out which major items are needed?

3. Do we register for baby gifts? If we do, do we register for just the basics or for all suggested items (or somewhere in between)?

Chapter 10: Expectations and Family of Origin

Expectations can create problems if they are not discussed. It is inevitable that life will change once you bring your baby home from the hospital. Take time to discuss how both of you see life once your baby is at home with you.

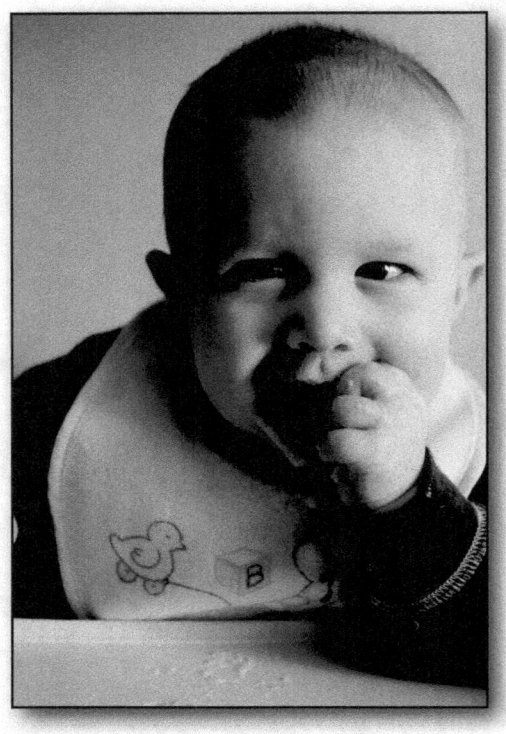

1. How do you see your role as a parent? How do you see your partner's role as a parent?

2. When you were growing up, how did you see your parents/guardians fitting into the role of parents? Do your expectations for your partner mirror your family of origin? Discuss the similarities and differences you both saw growing up.

3. Discuss how you see your relationship changing once a baby is brought into the relationship.

Chapter 11: Meeting the Baby's Needs

Since a baby cannot meet any of his or her own needs, the parents/guardians are now responsible for doing this. This can become overwhelming if all or most of the responsibility falls on one person. Each home is unique and each family has to find a schedule and routine that fits their situation. Discussing this prior to bringing the baby home will hopefully decrease tension, frustration, and anger.

1. Who will take care of giving the baby a bath (will this be one person's responsibility, will you take turns, will you have specific days of the week when it is one person's responsibility)?

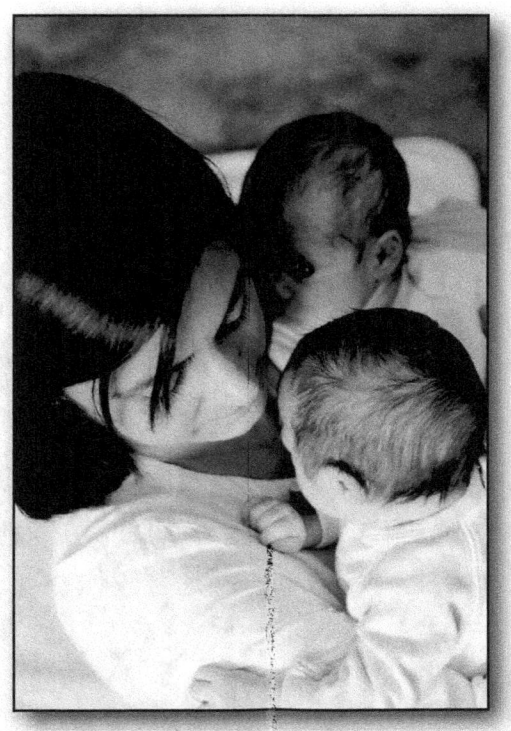

2. When the baby wakes in the middle of the night (sometimes more than once), how will you decide who will get out bed and feeds the baby?

3. If the baby cannot sleep and is up for an extended period of time in the middle of the night, who is going to stay up with the baby?

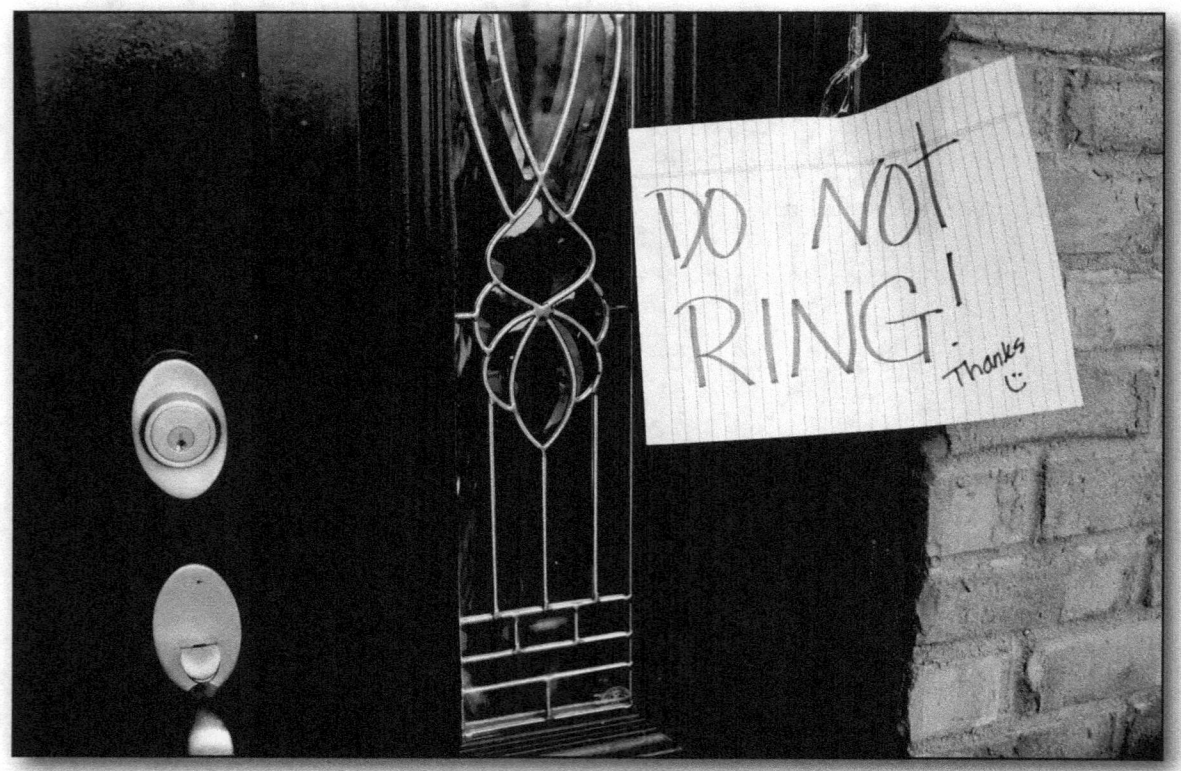

When a baby continually wakes through the night, it can be very exhausting for the parents. It may be beneficial to create a sleep schedule (for the parents). This schedule may block out a few hours each day for your partner to take a nap and then for your partner to let you nap.

Chapter 12: Parents' Anger and Frustration

Though babies are cute and cuddly, they can also be very demanding at very inconvenient times. It's important for parents to recognize when they are becoming angry or frustrated. Knowing how to manage your anger and frustration is key to keeping your baby safe.

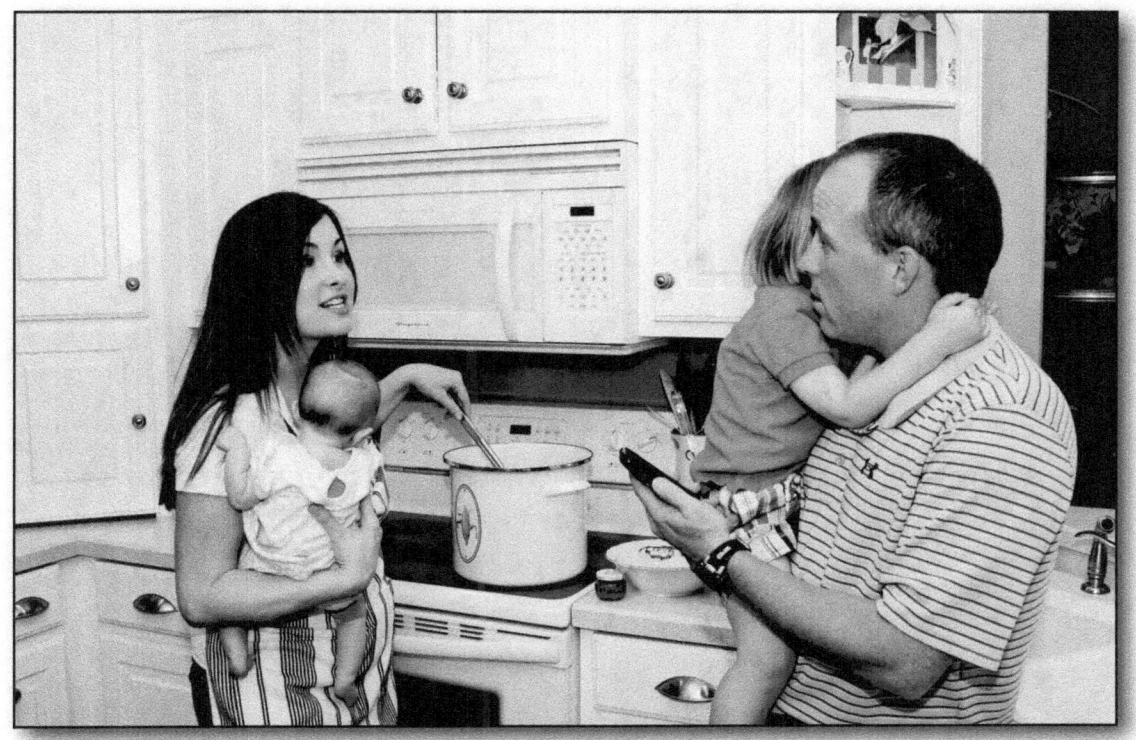

1. What physical signs do you show when you are becoming angry or frustrated? Ask your partner what signs he/she has noticed when you become angry or frustrated. Discuss a plan to help your partner when you notice he/she is becoming angry or frustrated.

2. Discuss the non-physical signs you experience when you become angry or frustrated (elevated temperature, pounding heart, negative thoughts, etc.). Discuss a plan of action you will take when you begin to notice these signs in yourself.

3. You may begin to feel anger or frustration when you are alone with the baby. What are some actions you can take to reduce your stress level (put the baby down in a safe place for a few minutes and walk away, call a friend, play some music, etc.)? It is very important that you are able to identify positive ways to release your negative emotions, both for your safety and for your baby.

4. What if you are unable to release your anger and frustration? Compile a list of other people you can call to help with the childcare and give you a small or large break.

Chapter 13: Visitors

Most of the time, family members want to visit the baby and are willing to help out with childcare, cleaning, and meals. This can be very helpful or very stressful if the family members are viewing this as a vacation or not offering to help where needed. This can also be a very sensitive issue when considering grandparents. It may be helpful to discuss the level of involvement you want from your extended family and discuss your decision with them, before coming home from the hospital.

1. Do you want family members to stay overnight at your house to help with your family's needs?

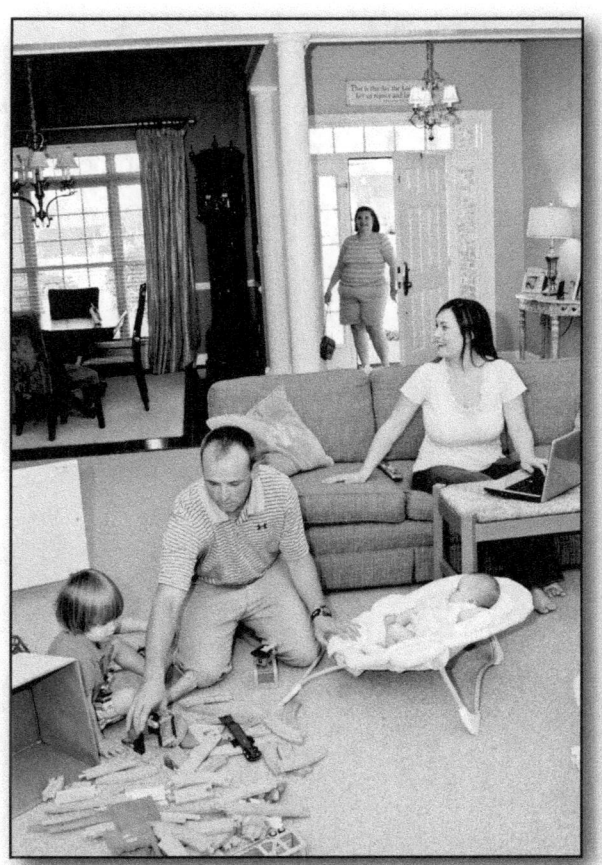

2. If family members are coming from out of town, and will be staying overnight, how soon do you want company?

3. When people come to visit, is there a time limit you want to put on visitors?

4. If family does come to visit for days or weeks to help your family, talk to them about what the type of help you need (childcare so parents can take naps, cooking meals, helping with cleaning, etc.).

Chapter 14: Relating to the Baby and Personality

Since everyone is different, you and your partner will probably relate to your baby differently. Personality, family of origin, and past experiences may influence your interactions with your child. Take some time to discuss the following topics.

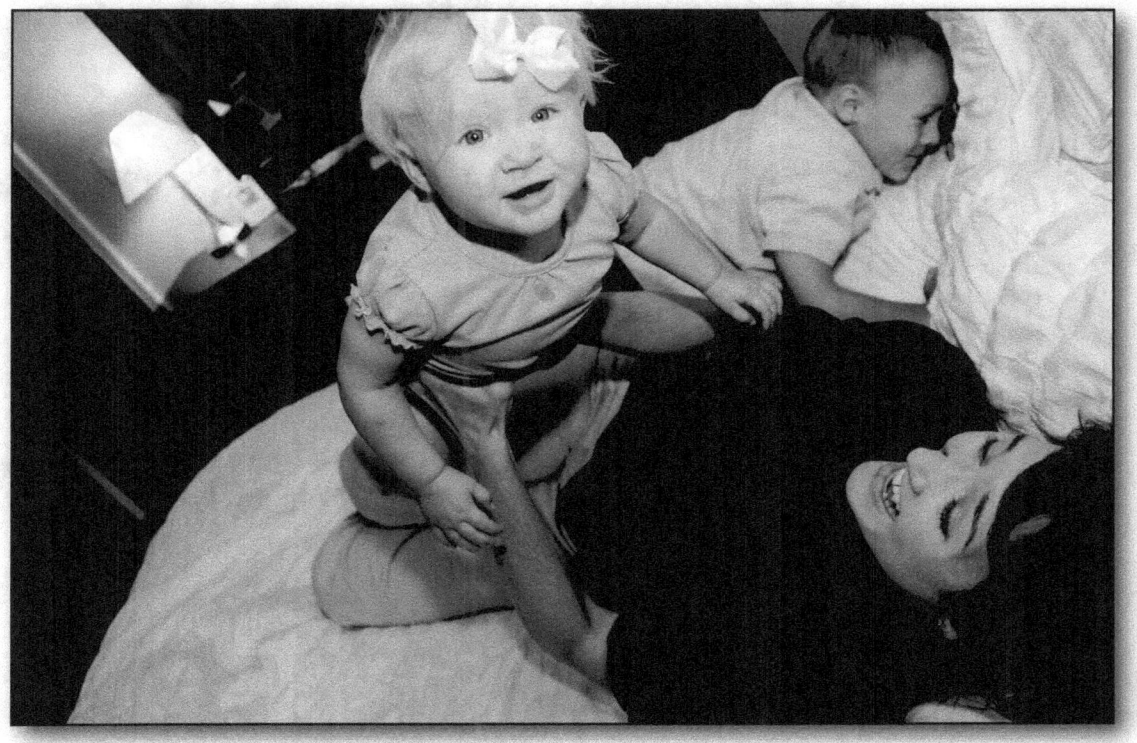

1. Are you the nurturing type?

2. Do you enjoy verbal or physical interaction more? Or are you the type that does not like much interaction and just enjoys being in the presence of others?

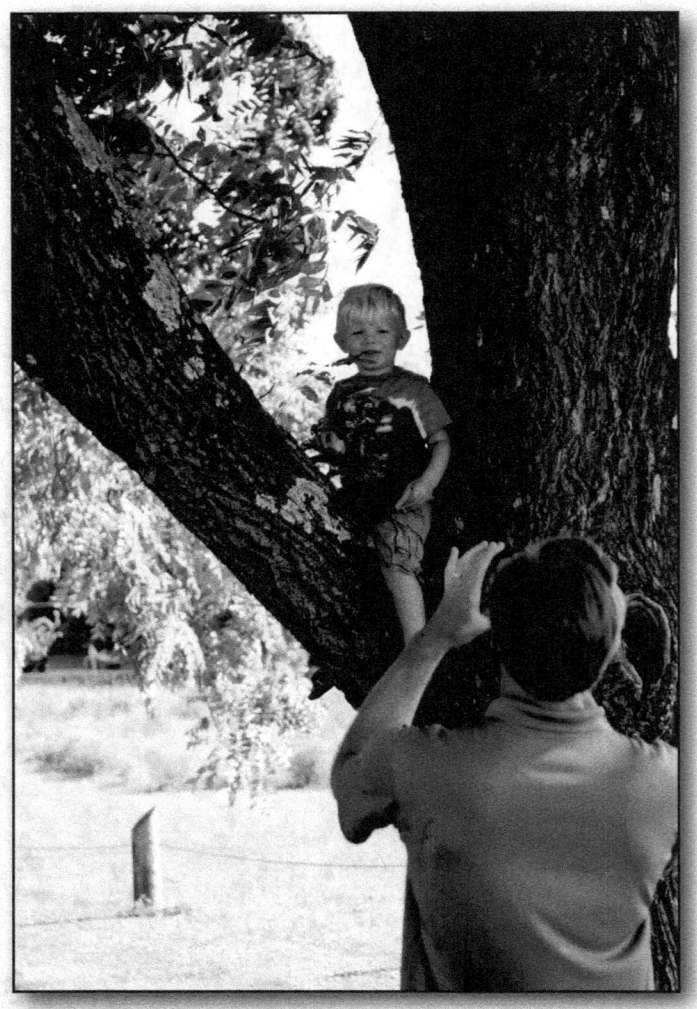

3. Are you easily angered?

4. How did you experience your parents/guardians interacting with you?

5. What would you like to do the same as your parents/guardians? What would you like to do differently?

6. Discuss the experiences in your life that have influenced your view of interactions between parent and child.

7. Discuss any concerns you may have regarding your mate's responses.

Chapter 15: Weeks After You are Home

What happens when the visitors have left your house, and you and your partner are on your own? Several sceneries may unfold at this time: one or both of you might be back at work, outside help may decrease or stop altogether, or the novelty of the baby may dwindle, to name just a few situations. This can be a difficult time for parents.

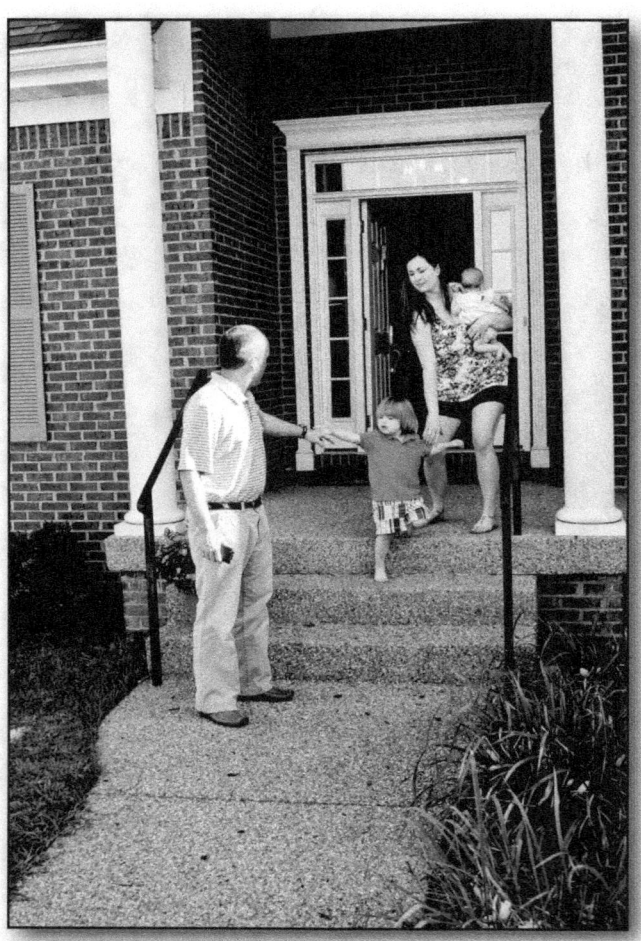

1.Discuss a plan of action you will take if you begin to feel "trapped" at home while your partner is at work, or you begin to resent your mate for getting out of the house. You may want to plan a break each day (find a parents' day out, play group, mommy and me class, etc.), and discuss your feelings with partner.

2. Sometimes the parent going back to work feels left out or resentful of the parent staying at home. How do you plan on working though these feelings if they arise (come home for lunch, set aside "guarded" time for you to spend with family, discuss feelings with partner, etc.)?

3. If both parents go back to work, there may be a struggle with guilt over leaving the child with someone else. Discuss your feelings about having someone else watch your child.

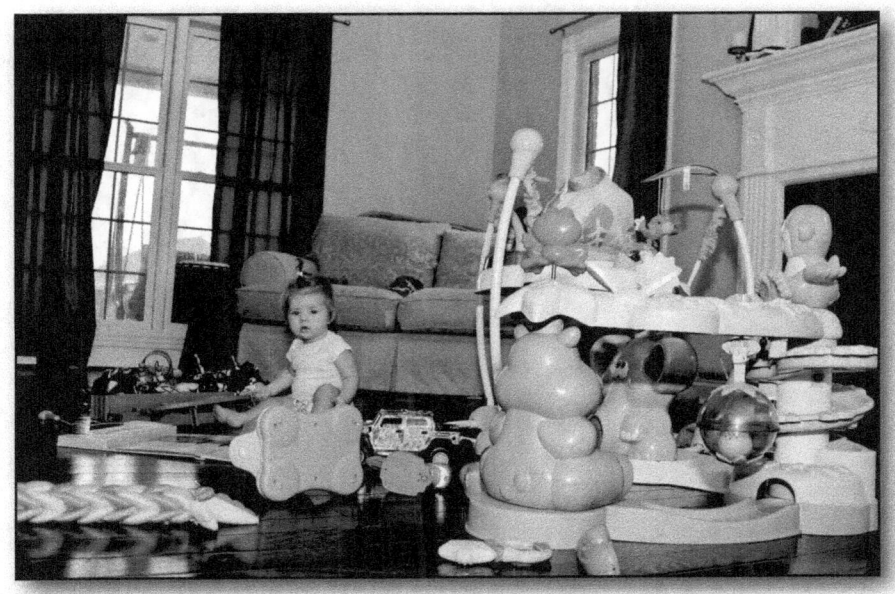

Authors Biography

Chandra Heath is a licensed marriage and family therapist in the state of Kentucky. Since 2002, Chandra has been working professionally with children, youth and families. After, she and her husband welcomed their second child into their family, Chandra became passionate about helping individuals and families transition and develop realistic expectations regarding pregnancy and caring for a baby.